Homemade Body Scrubs & Masks for Beginners

BY LINDSEY P

More than 50 Proven All Natural, Easy Recipes for Body Scrub & Facial Masks to Exfoliate, Nourish, & Care for Your Skin

2nd Edition

Table Of Contents

Introduction

I want to thank you and congratulate you for purchasing the book, *"Homemade Bodyscrubs & Masks for Beginners: More than 50 Proven all Natural, Easy Recipes for Body Scrubs & Facial Masks to Exfoliate, Nourish, & Care for Your Skin"*.

This book contains proven steps and strategies on how to create effective body scrubs and facial masks using a multitude of organic and natural products right out of your kitchen.

Exfoliation should always be a part of your skincare routine. This helps unclog your pores, slough off dull skin, balance sebum production, and even out your complexion. Importantly, exfoliation keeps the skin healthy, young-looking, and more glowing.

The good news is that you don't have to purchase expensive exfoliants and masks to have beautiful skin. You can easily make your own scrubs with the use of different items that are found in your home and garden. Use fruits in season or rummage in your kitchen cabinet and refrigerator and all the ingredients will surely be readily available. By creating your own skincare product, you can be sure that the ingredients are not just effective but safe and natural too. Try making these body scrubs and facial masks today!

Thanks again for purchasing this book, I hope you enjoy it!

Chapter 1: Benefits of Body Scrubbing and Facial Masks

The practice of scrubbing or exfoliating has been around for centuries. The ancient Egyptians were the first people to practice this. During the Middle Ages, people used wine with tartaric acid as a chemical exfoliant. Sounds painful? Not really. Tartaric acid naturally occurs in many plants and is even used for cooking. Scrubbing is still commonly practiced today in many different ways and for various reasons. Some exfoliate for aesthetic reasons while some do it for the sheer pleasure and relaxing feeling it gives them.

Beauty benefits

Our skin sheds constantly. The lower layer or the dermis constantly creates new skin which eventually migrates to the surface. When the skin reaches the surface, it is then worn out by the environment and physical activities. The worn out skin becomes dead skin cells that naturally shed off. The cycle of skin renewal takes about 30 days; so every month, dead skin cells die off and new cells emerge in the surface.

Sometimes however, the dead skin hardens and turns into calluses and causes the skin to feel rough and dry. Regular scrubbing can help the outer layer of the skin shed off more efficiently to give way to new skin cells that are smoother, whiter and look more youthful.

You might wonder, how often does a person shed skin and just how much dead skin cells are we talking about? Scientists estimate that a person has around 1.6 trillion skin cells. This is only an average estimate because the numbers will depend on the size of a person. An average person will shed around 30,000 to 40,000 skin cells per hour. This means that a person will shed about a million skin cells a day. That's about 3.6 kilograms of dead skin cells per year.

Sounds gross? Well here are more facts. The dead skin cells that are shed off become the dust in your house. See that picture frame that doesn't seem to run out of dust even though you clean it every day? The dust can actually come from dead skin cells being shed off. The more there are in the family living under one roof, the more chances of having dust, or rather dead skin cells, all over the house.

Gently scrubbing the skin regularly helps to enhance surface circulation. Normal friction on the skin does not shed all the dead skin cells, making the skin dull, flaky and ashy. Gentle exfoliation helps sweep away deep seated dirt and bacteria especially in non-exposed areas of the body.

How often should a person exfoliate?

Both beauty and health experts advise to exfoliate the body 2 to 3 times a week only. Just because the skin cells renew every 24 hours, it does not mean one needs to scrub every day. Too much scrubbing can make the skin look red and sore. It can even do more harm than good. Rubbing should be done gently in a circular motion. It is important to exfoliate both the skin on the face and the body in order to prevent dirt and bacteria buildup that might result to skin problems such as acne and boils.

What can I use to exfoliate my skin?

Most people do their scrubbing in the shower because it is much more convenient to rinse off the residue afterwards.

Most people use a loofah or a washcloth with a good body wash product. Special scrub mixtures such as those made from salt and sugar are usually done after a shower. Those are best used when the skin is already clean and still a bit wet. This will help the scrub mixture loosen up the dead skin cells.

After scrubbing, it is important to rinse thoroughly in order to remove all the granules that could possibly be left in the folds of the skin. The great thing about using an after-shower body scrub product is that it has special properties that can make the skin feel soft and supple. There's no need to use a moisturizing product such as oil or lotion after a scrub because the mixture will already leave the skin feeling moisturized and nourished.

Health benefits of scrubbing

Regular scrubbing can be therapeutic. Most body scrubs contain essential oils that give off a relaxing scent. Scrubbing in the shower will be like an aromatherapy session, reducing stress and anxiety. The gentle scrubbing motion on the skin is also similar to a massage, relaxing the muscles and providing an overall feeling of wellness and energy boost.

Regular scrubbing can improve circulation. When the skin is gently scrubbed in a circular motion, it improves the circulation of the blood on the outer layer of the skin. The tiny blood vessels closest to the skin called the capillaries are stimulated when the skin is subjected to friction. Stimulation can be as simple as rubbing the hands together to stimulate blood flow. Rubbing the body with a body scrub gives the same effect. When the capillaries are stimulated, it expands, resulting to better blood circulation. When the blood circulation on the skin is improved, the texture of the skin also improves.

Dangers of too much exfoliation

Regular scrubbing can help keep you clean and feeling smooth as a baby. However, too much scrubbing can actually be harmful. According to the U.S. Centers for Diseases Control and Prevention, people who wash and scrub too often than needed can be at risk of having *irritant contact dermatitis*. This is an inflammation of the skin caused either by chemicals or physical irritants. It can manifest as a rash and will feel more painful rather than itchy. Most health care professionals who use gloves and often need to wash their hands in order to prevent contamination often have this skin problem.

Our skin has an outermost skin barrier called the *stratum corneum*. When this barrier is breached, it often results to irritation, cracking, dryness and other forms of skin damage.

Benefits of using facial masks

Face masks are used to cleanse, moisturize, clarify, tighten skin and clear blemishes. But wait, isn't that what most facial wash, moisturizers and creams already promise to do? Why do we still need face masks? What can facial masks do that other beauty products can't? Some facial wash can strip the face of its natural oil and moisture. Moisturizers and creams can only nourish and help lighten skin. Facial masks target specific problem areas that some products can't.

Facial masks can help refine pores, unclogging it with oil and impurities to make the face cleaner and smoother. It also helps deeply moisturize skin without leaving the skin feeling blotchy and oily as what happens with some oil-based creams and moisturizers. Because the mask is left on the skin for several minutes, the skin soaks up the water from the mask, penetrating deeply, softening the skin and improving its elasticity. Face masks also help diminish fine lines and wrinkles, even out skin tone and firm the skin. If the skin looks tired, pale and dry, using a facial mask for several minutes can instantly make the skin look and feel soft, glowing and rejuvenated.

There are several types of facial masks. Some are in cream form, some in clay form and others are like sheet masks. One advantage of using cream-based masks is that you have control of the spot in the face where you want to put the mask. You can use it on the entire face or in the T-zone only, in the forehead only, or wherever the troubled spots are. When using a face mask, it is important to choose one that is made from ingredients that won't irritate the skin. There are different types of masks available for sensitive skin, acne-prone skin, oily skin and dry skin.

Face masks are very relaxing. Spas and beauty establishments that offer facial cleaning often use facial masks to help the patient relax and to further clean impurities and close the pores. After cleansing the face, a face mask will be applied and will be left to dry for at least 20 minutes before rinsing.

Facial masks are incredibly simple to use, even to make! Simply clean the face, put on the mask and wait for it to dry. When the skin already feels tight and dry, then the mask can be peeled and rinsed off. Facial masks can give an instant boost to the skin on the face, making it feel smooth and glowing after the treatment. This should be done at least once a week to help maintain the health and glow of the skin.

Facial masks may seem like a luxury beauty product, but it is actually very easy to do. In fact, do-it-yourself face masks are sometimes even better because you get to choose the freshest ingredients and these won't be as pricey as the store-bought products.

Chapter 2: Sugar Body Scrubs

The kitchen is the perfect place to concoct your ideal body scrub. Almost everything you need will be there, especially the most important ingredient – sugar. If you're on a diet and have sworn off all forms of sugar, don't throw those jars of sweet granules just yet. There's an even better use for it, and it won't be bad for your health.

Some people wonder why most body scrubs contain this sweet ingredient. It's because aside from the fact that the granules are perfect for exfoliating, it has properties that can do wonders for the skin.

Sugar is known as a natural humectant. This means that when added to another substance, it helps retain moisture. Sugar helps draw moisture and keep it locked into the skin. So products with sugar in it help hydrate and moisturize the skin.

Sugar is also a natural source of glycolic acid. This is an alpha hydroxyl acid (AHA) that helps break down skin cells in order for it to produce newer cells more efficiently. It is often used as an ingredient in products that are intended for treating age spots, wrinkles and sun damage. All AHAs help to exfoliate the outer layer of the skin so it is recommended to use sunscreen after application in order to protect the fresh newly exposed skin. Glycolic acid can irritate some skin types, therefore, concentrations are often only around 10 percent in most products.

Sugar scrub is most preferred compared to salt scrubs because it has finer granules that are gentler on the skin. Salt can be rough and coarse and can cause tiny tears on the skin.

Sugar is gentle enough to be used on the face. However, when making a sugar scrub for the face, choose brown sugar instead of the regular refined sugar because its granules are much softer. Brown sugar can be used by those who have sensitive skin. Raw sugar and refined sugar are generally used only for the body.

That being said, here's a list of some easy-to-do body scrub recipes made from sugar.

Banana & Sugar Scrub

Ingredients: 1 very ripe banana, ¼ teaspoon vanilla extract (pure), and 3 tablespoons granulated sugar

Directions: Combine all the ingredients together in a bowl. Mash the banana chunkily. Apply all over the body in a gentle, massaging motion. Rinse after 10-15 minutes.

Main ingredient: Banana

Bananas high Vitamin B6 and C content maintains and improves the elasticity of the skin. Its anti-oxidants also protect the skin from free radical damage and premature aging. It also helps hydrate the skin to make it suppler and prevent peeling.

Coconut Vanilla Sugar Scrub

Ingredients: ½ teaspoon fresh vanilla, ½ cup coconut oil, and ½ cup brown sugar

Mix all the ingredients together in a bowl or jar. Massage on your entire body for a few minutes before rinsing. You may also use the scrub as a massage cream.

Main Ingredient: coconut oil

Coconut oil is very effective in moisturizing and softening skin. Its antibacterial properties ward off bacteria and hasten healing. The antioxidants found in coconut oil also reduces appearance of wrinkles, thwart cellular aging.

Peppermint Coco Scrub

Ingredients: ½ cup coconut oil, 1 cup sugar, 1 tablespoon powdered milk, 2 drops peppermint essential oil, and 2-3 drops green food coloring (optional)

Directions: Combine all the ingredients, except the oil, in a container. Mix well. Add in the peppermint essential oil and stir thoroughly. Massage into the skin for a few minutes. Rinse with warm water.

Main ingredients: coconut oil and peppermint essential oil

Coconut oil helps moisturize and hydrate the skin to keep it supple and young- looking. Peppermint essential oil is cool and very refreshing. It revitalizes dull skin and removes excess oil to keeps back acne at bay.

Lavender Vanilla Scrub

Ingredients: ½ cup melted coconut oil, 4 tablespoons sweet almond oil, 15 drops lavender essential oil, 1 teaspoon fresh vanilla, and 1 cup white sugar

Directions: Transfer the sugar into a bowl. Mix in the sweet almond oil and coconut oil. Next, stir in the lavender essential oil and vanilla. Massage the scrub all over the body. Leave on for 20 to 30 minutes before rinsing with warm water.

Main ingredient: lavender essential oil

Lavender essential oil's scent effectively soothes and calms the mind and body. This essential oil also has antiseptic properties that heals acne and wounds, minimizes redness and swelling, and reduces appearance of scars. It also increases blood circulation, firms the skin, and relieves sore muscles and cramps.

Cinna-Choco Scrub

Ingredients: ½ cup white sugar, 1 cup brown sugar, ½ tablespoon cocoa powder, ½ tablespoon cinnamon powder, and 2 tablespoons olive oil.

Directions: Combine all the ingredients in a bowl and stir well. Apply on the skin and massage in a circular motion. Rinse with warm water.

Main ingredient: cocoa powder

Cocoa powder is full of anti-oxidants that help protect the skin from free radical damage. Its natural exfoliants also remove dead skin cells to achieve a more glowing complexion.

Citrusy Fresh Scrub

Ingredients: 20 drops lime essential oil, 3 drops orange essential oil, 5 drops lemon essential oil, 3 drops bergamot essential oil, 1/3 cup melted virgin coconut oil, ½ cup carrier oil (jojoba oil or safflower oil), and 2 cups sugar

Directions: Except for the carrier oil, stir all the ingredients in the bowl. Slowly add the carrier oil into the mixture until you've reached the appropriate consistency. Massage unto the skin and rinse thoroughly.

Main ingredient: lemon and lime essential oils

Lemon and lime essential oils both have astringent, antibacterial, and antiseptic properties. It is quite effective in reducing sebum production and preventing and treating acne. These essential oils also have anti-aging properties to reduce appearance of wrinkles and maintain a youthful glow.

Sugar Coffee Scrub

Ingredients: ¼ cup ground coffee, ¼ cup raw brown sugar, 2 tablespoons virgin coconut oil, 1 tablespoon olive oil, and 1 tablespoon sea salt

Directions: Combine all the ingredients thoroughly. Grab a handful of the scrub and massage your body in a circular motion for several minutes. Rinse with warm water.

Main ingredient: ground coffee

Ground coffee effectively reduces the appearance of cellulite. This is because the antioxidants and caffeine in the coffee increases blood circulation in the body and dilates the blood vessels. The grounds also exfoliate the skin to make it luminous and supple.

Coco Ginger Scrub

Ingredients: 1 tablespoon coarsely chopped peeled ginger root, ¼ cup sunflower oil, ¼ cup coconut oil, ¼ cup kosher salt, ¾ cup granulated sugar, and 4 drops lemongrass essential oil

Directions: Using a small pan, heat ginger and coconut oil

over a low flame for 10 minutes. This will allow the oils and scent of the ginger to mix with the oil. Turn off the heat and filter the liquid into a bowl. Discard the ginger bits.

Mix in the sunflower oil into the warm ginger-infused oil. Stir well and add the salt and sugar. Stir and add the lemongrass essential oil. Massage this scrub all over the body and leave on for 5 minutes. Rinse as usual.

Main ingredient: ginger root

A favorite home remedy, ginger root possesses anti-inflammatory properties that help heal a variety of skin diseases, prevent acne, reduce swelling, and stop redness. Its antioxidant properties also make the skin tight, glowing, and energized.

Easy Vanilla Sugar Scrub

Ingredients: ¼ cup white sugar, ½ cup brown sugar, ¼ cup sweet almond oil, and 3 tablespoons vanilla extract

Directions: Combine the brown and white sugars in a mixing bowl. Add the sweet almond oil and vanilla extract. Stir well. Apply the body scrub on damp skin and massage for several minutes until the sugars dissolve. Rinse with warm water.

Main ingredient: vanilla extract

Not just used for baked goods, vanilla is chockfull of antioxidants, vitamins and minerals. It improves your skin tone, hastens wound healing, soothes irritated skin, and prevents premature aging.

Spice-y Scrub

Ingredients: ¾ cup almond oil, 2 teaspoons ginger powder, 2 teaspoons cinnamon powder, 2 teaspoons nutmeg powder, 1 cup granulated sugar, and 1 cup brown sugar

Directions: Put all the dry ingredients first in a bowl. Add the oil and whisk together thoroughly. Massage into the skin and rinse after a several minutes.

Main ingredients: ginger, cinnamon, and nutmeg

Ginger naturally prevents premature skin aging, reduces appearance of wrinkles and sagging skin, fights infections, calms swelling, and purifies and smoothens the skin. Cinnamon contains antimicrobial and antiseptic properties that aid in fighting infections and warding off bad odor. Nutmeg helps reduce blackheads and makes scars lighter and less noticeable. It also offers relief from muscle and joint pain.

Reviving Vanilla Scrub

Ingredients: juice of 3 lemon, 15 vanilla beans, 9 drops vanilla essential oil, and 9 tablespoons brown sugar.

Directions: Get your vanilla beans and slice them lengthwise to open. Use a spoon to scrape out the seeds and transfer to a mixing bowl. Add in the lemon juice and stir. Mix in the brown sugar and essential oil. Stir well. Apply the scrub on the body and massage well. Rinse with warm water and follow with cold water.

Main ingredient: vanilla essential oil

Vanilla is always a favorite when it comes to soothing scents but its benefits go beyond its fragrance. Vanilla contains anti-inflammatory components that stop and soothe swelling. Its antibacterial properties kill acne and body odor causing bacteria, boost wound healing, and reduce infections.

Vitamin Lavender Scrub

Ingredients: 1 tablespoon Vitamin E, 3 tablespoons almond oil, ½ cup coconut oil (organic), and 1/3 cup Celtic sea salt, 1 cup cane sugar (organic), and lavender essential oil

Directions: Combine the salt and sugar in a bowl. Add in the coconut oil and almond oil. Mix well. Stir in the vitamin E and the 9 drops of lavender essential oil. Scrub on wet skin and rinse with warm water after a few minutes.

Main ingredients: lavender and vitamin E

Lavender is widely used for its calming and cleansing properties. It helps stop itching and swelling caused by insect bites and stings, minor burns, and minor wound bleeding. Vitamin E is a powerful antioxidant that stops premature skin aging and further cell damage. It promotes younger looking skin that's supple and healthy.

Milk Body Scrub

Ingredients: 2 tablespoons fresh whole milk, 2 tablespoons light vegetable oil, ½ cup granulated white sugar

Directions: Combine all the ingredients in a bowl. Mix well until creamy. Rub on damp skin and leave on for 25-30 minutes. Rinse with warm water.

Main ingredient: milk

Milk improves skin complexion by making it fairer, brighter, and softer. It also cleanses the skin while reducing the size of the pores. Milk naturally restores the skin's moisture to keep it supple and young-looking.

Spicy Sugar Scrub

Ingredients: ¾ cup sugar, 2 tablespoons fresh orange zest, 2 tablespoons ground cloves, 1 tablespoon dried rose petals, and 1 ½ cups sesame oil

Directions: Using a bowl, mix all the ingredients thoroughly. Apply on damp skin and massage for several minutes. Rinse well.

Main ingredient: ground cloves

Ground cloves reduce inflammation symptoms and provide a mild anesthetic effect to subdue body and muscle pain.

Matcha Sugar Scrub

Ingredients: 1 teaspoon matcha green tea powder, 1 tablespoon green tea (from tea bags), 1 cup granulate sugar, ½ cup coconut oil

Directions: Combine all the ingredients together in a bowl. Massage on damp skin for several minutes before rinsing.

Main ingredient: green tea

Full of antioxidants, green tea firms and tones the skin to make it look younger. It fights redness and irritation from

various skin diseases like rosacea, psoriasis or eczema.

Pumpkin Pie Spice Sugar Scrub

Ingredients: 1 cup brown sugar, ½ teaspoon pumpkin pie spices, ½ teaspoon Vitamin E oil, ½ cup coconut oil

Directions: Combine all of the ingredients in a mixing bowl. It can be stored in a jar with a tight lid to keep away moisture. This recipe can last up to 2 months if stored properly. It can be used on the face and body, especially on the feet.

Main ingredient: pumpkin pie

Pumpkin is rich in beta-carotene and antioxidants that combat free radicals that are responsible for poor skin tone. It also contains Vitamin C. It helps reduce the risk of sunburn and even helps fight acne.

Aloe Vera Scrub

Ingredients: 1 cup white cane sugar, 1 cup vegetable glycerine, aloe vera gel (just a small amount), 1-2 drops of essential oil (optional).

Directions: Combine all ingredients in a bowl until everything is mixed thoroughly. Scoop a small amount and rub onto skin. The mixture will dry a little and make the skin feel tight. Leave on for around 3 minutes before rinsing.

Main ingredient: aloe vera

Aloe Vera is known as a wonder gel when it comes to skin care. It can cure sunburn, treat acne, act as a moisturizer, fight aging, and lessen stretch mark visibility.

Shea Butter Body Scrub

Ingredients: ½ cup of raw Shea butter, 2/3 cup sugar. 1/3 cup olive oil, 1/8 teaspoon Vitamin E oil, 10 drops of preferred essential oil

Directions: Beat Shea butter in a large bowl until it turns into a creamy texture. This should take around 5 minutes. Add the olive oil and vitamin E gradually and mix thoroughly. Lastly, stir in the sugar and essential oil. Store mixture in a tight jar. Massage onto skin in a circular motion. Rinse off with warm water.

Main ingredient: Shea butter

Shea butter is known to provide relief for many skin ailments, from minor problems to the most troublesome. It is great for moisturizing dry skin, treating sunburn, reducing scars and blemishes, evening out skin tone, relieving itchy skin due to dryness, healing small skin wounds, and for lessening and preventing stretch marks, for minor burns, eczema and a lot more!

Coconut Coffee Body Scrub

Ingredients: ½ cup ground coffee, ½ cup coconut palm sugar, ¼ cup coconut oil, 1 teaspoon ground cinnamon

Directions: Mix all ingredients together until thoroughly blended. Coconut oil tends to solidify in cold temperature so it might be necessary to melt it slightly before mixing it in with the other ingredients.

Main ingredient: ground coffee, coconut oil, cinnamon

Coffee is rich in antioxidants and can also treat

inflammation. *Coconut oil is filled with vitamins and minerals that do wonders for the skin, aside from its intense moisturizing properties. Cinnamon helps get rid of bacteria and improves circulation.*

Coconut and Rose Body Scrub

Ingredients: coconut oil, raw cane sugar or ordinary brown sugar, rose petals, almond or jojoba oil, an airtight jar

Directions: Take note that there's no particular portion or measurements of the ingredients in this recipe. Just put an approximate amount that you think will fit into the jar. Layer all of the ingredients in the jar. Start by placing a large scoop of coconut oil (assuming that the oil is in solid state) in the jar. Place a bunch of rose petals on top of the oil. Place several tablespoons of sugar on top of the rose petals. Pour a small amount of almond or jojoba oil on the sugar.

Wait a few minutes until the oil seeps down to reach the rose petals. Add a little more oil if necessary. Cover the mixture and store in this state to allow all the ingredients to infuse and for the petals to be soaked and softened by the oil. When ready to use, take a spoon and mash all the ingredients together. Rub the skin in a circular motion and wash with warm water.

Main ingredient: rose petals

The ancient Romans use rose petals to make perfumed baths, but it does more than provide an aromatic bath. Apparently, roses have antifungal, antibacterial and antiviral properties. This makes it an ideal solution for skin problems such as sunburn, healing minor cuts, and other skin conditions.

Chapter 3: Salt Body Scrubs

Salt scrubs are commonly used in the beauty industry because their granules are safe and ideal for making body scrubs. Sea salts or Epsom salts are used because these contain minerals and have properties that are beneficial for the skin. Epsom salt for example, contains magnesium that can reduce skin inflammation, and sulfates that help to remove toxins from the skin. The salts, when mixed with oil and applied to skin, give a gentle abrasive action that improves circulation of blood in the capillaries and invigorates the skin. Salt also has antiseptic properties that kill bacteria and relieve symptoms such as itching and pain which is associated with skin problems caused by bacterial infections.

It helps unclog pores and removes hardened dead skin cells, giving the skin a natural glow after the scrub. When the dead skin cells are removed, it encourages regeneration of new skin and gives way for the cells to produce new, healthy and smoother cells. New skin cells will look more youthful, tighter and firmer. Salt scrubs also even out skin tones and reduce discoloration.

How to choose salt for the scrub?

There's really no need to use fancy salts in a salt scrub; in fact, you can simply use ordinary table salt! But if you are looking for a more luxurious feel, you can use finely textured sea salts found locally. In most groceries and beauty stores, there will be packages of dead sea salts or bath salts. Some grinding may be required in order for you to get the consistency you want.

Kosher salts have a much larger grain but it will work especially for stubborn and hardened skin cells. The great thing about salt is that it is extremely affordable, even more than sugar. So stock up on these wonderful salt scrubs. It would only cost pennies compared to store-bought products and they work just as wonderful.

Here's a list of easy-to-do salt scrub recipes for you to enjoy!

Coarse Lavender Salt Scrub

Ingredients: 1/3 cup grapeseed oil, 1 tablespoon dried lavender,16 drops lavender essential oil, and ½ cup coarse sea salt

Directions: Put the sea salt in a mixing bowl and pour in the grapeseed oil. Stir the ingredients together. Mix in the dried lavender. Add the essential oil and combine well. Apply on wet skin and massage gently. Do not use this scrub if you have any open wounds or cuts.

Main ingredient: lavender

When used in aromatherapy, the scent of lavender eliminates stress and anxiety. If applied on the skin, it offers an analgesic and sedative effect that eliminates minor aches and pains. Lavender's astringent properties minimize swelling too.

Thyme Lemon Salt Scrub

Ingredient: 2 teaspoons fresh thyme leaves, zest of a whole lemon, ½ cup organic almond oil, and 1 cup plain kosher salt

Directions: Pour the salt in a bowl. Add in the thyme leaves and lemon zest. Mix in the almond oil. Combine all ingredients thoroughly. Massage on damp skin and leave on for 20 minutes before rinsing with warm water.

Main ingredients: thyme and lemon

Thyme is very beneficial to the skin. It helps reduce inflammation, heals lesions, and kills acne-causing bacteria. Lemon is also equally beneficial because it brightens the skin, reduces age spots, makes blackheads disappear, and stop excess oil production.

Tea Tree Salt Scrub

Ingredients: 3 teaspoons 15% tea tree oil and 1 cup kosher salt

Directions: Place a kosher salt in a bowl. Add in the tea tree oil and mix well. Apply on wet skin and massage gently. Leave on for several minutes and rinse. If using on dry skin, add a few drops of water to a handful of scrub and apply. Leave on until dry and brush off.

Main ingredient: tea tree oil

Tea tree oil contains anti-inflammatory properties that treat acne and inflamed skin allergies. Its anti-bacterial components can cure athlete's foot, skin dandruff, and other bacterial skin ailments.

Sage Salt Scrub

Ingredients: 4-7 fresh sage leaves, ½ cup date sugar, 1 cup olive oil, fresh zest of 1 grapefruit, and 2 cups fine sea salt

Directions: Place the sage and olive oil in the blender and process on high. Transfer the pureed mixture in a bowl and add the date sugar and sea salt. Stir well. Add the grapefruit zest and mix thoroughly. Apply the scrub on the skin and massage for two minutes. Rinse well.

Main ingredient: sage leaves

Sage leaves extract are often added to many skin care products because of their efficacy. Rich in vitamin A and calcium, it helps in daily cell regeneration to stop premature aging and wrinkles. It also improves blood circulation in the body to reduce varicose veins and cellulite. Sage also hastens healing of skin disorders including psoriasis and eczema symptoms.

Citrus Salt Scrub

Ingredients: 6 tablespoons iodized salt, 2 tablespoons Epsom salt, 2 cups white sugar, citrus essential oil (grapefruit, sweet orange, or lemon), and 1 cup jojoba oil

Directions: Put the salt and sugar inside the blender or food processor. Pulse several times to make the crystals finer. Transfer the mixture in a bowl. Add the jojoba oil and whisk to combine. Add about 25-30 drops of the citrus essential oil and mix. Use on this scrub on wet skin. Massage in circular motions and rinse well.

Main ingredient: Epsom salt and citrus essential oil

A popular natural remedy, Epsom salt contains magnesium and sulfate that reduces inflammation, improves muscle function, flushes out toxins, and increases nutrient absorption. Citrus essential oils are wide used for their light and refreshing aromas. Their scent uplifts the mood and energizes the body. When applied on the skin, it helps fight acne and prevent oily skin.

Scented Epsom Scrub

Ingredients: 1 cup Epsom salt, 1 cup sweet almond oil, and 10 drops rose essential oil

Directions: Combine all the ingredients in a small bowl. Mix well until a thick texture is achieved. Scrub all over your wet skin and massage gently. Rinse well and pat to dry.

Main ingredient: rose essential oil

Rose essential oil is commonly used in many skin care products because of its appealing scent. Apart from this, the oil also reduces appearance of stretch marks and scars, regenerates healthy skin cells, moisturizes very dry skin, and heals symptoms of eczema.

Salt Floral Scrub

Ingredients: 1 cup sea salt, 1 tablespoon dried rose, 7 drops rose hip seed oil, and ½ cup sweet almond oil

Directions: Mix the salt and oils in the bowl. Add in the dried rose and crush gently. Apply on the skin and massage for several minutes. Rinse well.

Main ingredient: dried rose

Dried rose contains beta carotene and B vitamins that help keeps skin fresh, moisturized, and healthy. It also reduces swelling and fights various skin infections.

Pumpkin Scrub

Ingredients: ½ cup pure pumpkin puree, 1 cup sea salt, 1 tablespoon sweet almond oil, and 1 teaspoon honey.

Directions: Mix the all the ingredients together. If you want the mixture to be oilier, add more almond oil.

Main ingredient: pumpkin puree

Perfect for all skin types, pumpkin contains a lot of vitamins that aid in healing, stopping free radical damage, and alleviating skin dryness. Its enzymes and anti-oxidants nourish the skin while removing dead skin cells.

Ultimate Sea Salt Scrub

Ingredients: 1 cup coarse sea salt, ½ cup baby oil or vegetable oil

Directions: Combine all ingredients in a bowl and then cover it. Let the mixture sit for 24 hours. Stir the mixture and its ready to use. Apply on skin in a circular motion and then rinse.

Main ingredient: sea salt

Sea salt is excellent for detoxifying the skin and getting rid of impurities. It also has antiseptic effect and increases circulation.

Exfoliating Oatmeal Scrub

Ingredients: ½ cup fine sea salt, ¼ cup ground uncooked oatmeal, ¼ cup flaxseed oil, ¼ cup extra virgin olive oil, 8 drops of geranium oil

Directions: Mix all the ingredients together and store in a sealed glass jar. This scrub is best used after shower. Scrub all over the body then rinse.

Main ingredient: oatmeal

Oatmeal is great for skin protection as it helps maintain the skin's natural barrier to guard against the harsh environmental pollution and chemicals. It helps moisturize the skin and improves collagen deposition.

Fragrant Salt Scrub

Ingredients: 3 cups fine sea salt, ¾ cup extra virgin olive oil, ¾ cup sweet almond oil, and your choice of essential oil

Directions: Mix the all the ingredients together in a bowl. Once thoroughly mixed, store it in a sealed glass jar. Use this scrub after showering. Scrub all over the body then rinse.

Main ingredient: almond oil

Almond oil helps lighten dark spots, gets rid of the skin's impurities and loosens dead skin cells. It also helps ease symptoms of eczema and psoriasis.

Lavender Salt Scrub

Ingredients: ¼ cup fine sea salt, ¼ cup extra virgin olive oil, 3 to 5 drops of lavender essential oil

Directions: Mix all the ingredients together in a bowl. The scrub is best used after a shower. Add a little bit of water or liquid soap when using the scrub. Rinse thoroughly after scrubbing.

Main ingredient: lavender

The scent of lavender essential oil while scrubbing helps provide a soothing and relaxing feeling, almost like an aromatherapy massage. It will help ease stress and give an

uplifting feeling. It has antiseptic properties that help heal minor wounds, fight acne, prevent wrinkles, tone the skin, and heal sunburn.

Peppermint Foot Scrub

Ingredients: 1 ½ cup fine sea salt, 1/3 cup extra virgin olive oil, 3 drops of peppermint essential oil

Directions: Mix all the ingredients together and store in a dry, clean container with cover. This mixture is best used after a foot bath or foot soak. It gently exfoliates callused soles and heels.

Main ingredient: peppermint

Peppermint essential oil has antibacterial properties that stop the growth of different kinds of bacteria in the body. It also has antifungal properties. It has long been used as an effective treatment for common skin ailments such as rashes. The menthol in peppermint also helps prevent oil production that's why it is often used in beauty products that are intended for those with oily or greasy skin.

Lemon and Thyme Salt Scrub

Ingredients: 1 cup kosher salt, ½ cup pure organic almond oil, lemon zest (1 lemon), 2 teaspoons of fresh thyme with leaves stripped off from the stems

Directions: Place the salt in a container then add in the lemon zest and thyme. Add in the almond oil and stir. This mixture is best used in the shower. If stored in an airtight container, this mixture can last up to 6 months.

Main ingredient: lemon and thyme

Lemon is commonly used to treat pigmentation problems, pimples, and helps soften the skin. Thyme is known to contain antioxidants and also works as a natural astringent for the skin.

Coconut Salt Scrub

Ingredients: 1 cup sea salt, ½ cup coconut oil, ¼ cup vitamin E oil, 2 to 3 drops of essential oil

Directions: Simply mix all the ingredients in a clean bowl. Store in an airtight container.

Main ingredient: coconut oil

Coconut oil is known as the wonder oil for its multitude of health benefits. It has antibacterial properties that can treat acne and other skin problems. It has anti-aging properties, moisturizes, cleans, and acts as sunscreen.

Chapter 4: Salt and Sugar Free Body Scrubs

Ran out of salt and sugar in the kitchen? Don't fret. It is still possible to create a luscious body scrub without these two popular ingredients. You just need something coarse to replace them such as oatmeal, almond meal or nuts. Will the result still be as effective without these two basic ingredients? The answer is yes, and for some people, even more favorable. Everyone have different types of skin. Therefore, some people yield more positive results to body scrubs that contain other ingredients such as oatmeal, almonds and other fruits and vegetables. Check out some of the recipes below, try them out and see if these will also work for you. These recipes are best for all types of skin.

Here are some salt and sugar free body scrub recipes your body will surely love!

Oatmeal Chamomile Scrub

Ingredients: 4 tablespoons ground almonds, 1 tablespoon cornstarch, 4 tablespoons oatmeal, 1 tablespoon chamomile flowers, 2 tablespoons sweet almond oil, and 5 drops lavender extract

Directions: Place the ground almonds, cornstarch and oatmeal in a spice grinder or blender. Add the chamomile flowers and process well. Mix in the sweet almond oil and lavender extract. Stir well. To use, get a handful of the scrub and add several drops of water. Massage on damp skin for several minutes and wash off with warm water.

Main ingredient: ground almonds and chamomile flowers

Almonds are rich in phytochemicals that treat pimples, acne, and other skin conditions. It also reduces sebum production and prevents overly oily skin. Chamomile's anti-inflammatory and antiseptic properties soothe skin redness and swelling brought upon by acne, eczema, and minor burns.

Firming Scrub

Ingredients: 2 egg whites, 2 bay leaves, 1 celery stalk, ½ cup unpeeled cucumber slices, ¼ cup wheat germ, ½ cup hearts of palm (chopped), ¼ cup full-fat powdered milk, ¼ unpeeled russet potato slices, 1 teaspoon mint leaves, 1 teaspoon coconut extract, and 1 teaspoon vanilla extract

Ingredients: Place all the ingredients in a blender. Process until all the contents takes on a thick consistency. Apply all over the body and massage for several minutes. Leave on for 20 minutes before rinsing with lukewarm water.

Main ingredient: russet potato, and celery

Russet potatoes naturally brighten the skin's complexion, refresh tired skin, remove dark spots, and nourish very dry skin. It also prevent acne, heal insect stings and bites, and soothe minor burns. Celery contains powerful antioxidants that delay skin aging, protect from free radical damage, and hydrates from the inside out. It also maintains the skin luminosity and elasticity.

Honey Wheat Germ Scrub

Ingredients: 2 tablespoons clear honey, 1 tablespoon wheat germ, 1 teaspoon sunflower oil, and 1 teaspoon fresh lemon juice

Directions: In small bowl, combine the wheat germ and the honey. Add the sunflower oil and lemon juice to the mixture. Stir well. Scrub on damp skin for several minutes. Rinse thoroughly.

Main ingredient: wheat germ

Wheat germ is rich in zinc which helps in skin cell production. It also contains anti-inflammatory properties that stop symptoms of eczema and other skin diseases and lessen acne swelling.

Almond Meal Scrub

Ingredients: ½ cup ground almond meal,1/2 cup oats (finely ground oats), and rosewater

Directions: Place the oats and almonds in the blender. Process them until well-combined. Transfer into a small bowl. Gently pour in the rosewater drop by drop until a paste is formed. Apply on damp skin and massage for several minute. Leave on skin for 30 minutes before rinsing.

Main ingredient: almond meal

Almond meal helps smoothen and soften the skin and removes dead skin cells. It also reduces swelling and clarifies skin complexion.

Coffee, Honey and Coconut Oil Scrub

Ingredients: 1 cup coffee grounds, ½ cup honey, 1 cup coconut oil

Directions: Mix all the ingredients together thoroughly until it turns into a paste-like consistency. Use the mixture in the shower. Massage onto skin and leave on for a few minutes before rinsing with warm water. Use a moisturizer after shower to lock in the moisture.

Main ingredient: coffee, honey, coconut oil

Coconut oil is best for hydrating the skin while the coffee grounds mixed with the honey work best for exfoliation. This mixture will help the skin remove flakiness and give it an afterglow.

Grapefruit and Oatmeal Body Scrub

Ingredients: 1 fresh grapefruit, 2 tablespoons oatmeal

Directions: Squeeze out the pulp and juice of the grapefruit and put it in a bowl. Add in the oatmeal and mix until it turns into a smooth paste. You can add in more oatmeal or juice in order to get the consistency you desire. Scrub the paste-like mixture on the face and on the body. Leave on for a few minutes before rinsing.

Main ingredient: grapefruit, oatmeal

The grapefruit contains citrus that helps stimulate the skin and aids in exfoliation. The coarseness of the oatmeal provides a gentle exfoliation while hydrating the skin.

Baking Soda and Oatmeal Scrub

Ingredients: 2 heaping tablespoons of oatmeal, 1 teaspoon of baking soda, water

Directions: Mix the two ingredients together. Gradually add in small amounts of water until the mixture turns into a sticky paste. This recipe will only make a small amount of scrub. Double or triple the ingredients if you desire to make more. Massage the mixture in the face and body in a circular motion. Let it sit for a few minutes before rinsing.

Main ingredient: Baking soda

Baking soda is ideal for exfoliation because it is not too coarse and therefore helps to gently exfoliate the top layer of the dead skin cells. It is also safe to use even on sensitive skin.

Apple Cider Oatmeal Scrub

Ingredients: 8 tablespoons oatmeal, 1 tablespoon apple cider, 1 tablespoon dark organic honey, 2 teaspoons ground almonds

Directions: Warm the honey until it becomes a little runny or watery, but not too hot so it won't burn. Place the melted honey in a bowl and add in all the other ingredients. Mix everything until it turns into a smooth paste. Rub the mixture on the skin in a circular motion and leave on for 10 to 15 minutes. Rinse with alternating warm and cold water, but end it in a splash of cold water to close the pores.

Main ingredient: apple cider

Apple cider vinegar has long been used for treating warts, acne and other skin problems. It also has antibacterial properties that can help rid the skin of common problems associated with bacterial infection.

Cucumber Yogurt Scrub

Ingredients: ¼ medium peeled cucumber, 2 tablespoons plain unflavored yogurt (with active cultures), 2 tablespoons oatmeal, 1 teaspoon jojoba, 1 teaspoon sweet almond oil

Directions: Cut the cucumber into small pieces and put them in a blender or food processor to liquefy. Add in the rest of the ingredients to the food processor or blender and whisk until the mixture turns into a smooth paste. Rub onto body and face in a circular motion then rinse with alternating warm and cold water.

Main ingredient: cucumber, yogurt

Cucumber is best known for reducing eye bags and removing dark circles under the eye. Other benefits on skin include treating sunburn, tightening pores, and reducing freckles. Yogurt, when eaten is packed with nutrients such as zinc, calcium and B-vitamins. But it also helps tighten skin pores and remove acne.

Avocado-Almond Scrub

Ingredients: 1 cup oatmeal, 1 tablespoon ground Almonds, 1 ripe avocado (peeled)

Directions: Mix the oatmeal and almonds and then set aside. Mash the peeled avocado to a pulp. Using a clean washcloth, grab some of the avocado pulp then dip it in the almond and oatmeal mixture. Rub onto skin in a circular motion to exfoliate. Rinse thoroughly and tone and moisturize afterwards.

Main ingredient: avocado

Avocado is rich in antioxidants plus vitamins A and C. It is used to moisturize not only the skin but also the hair.

Chapter 5: Facial Masks for All Skin Types

If you want to make a homemade facial mask to give away as a gift, it is best to make one that is ideal for all skin types. Generally, these types of facial masks are easy to do and the ingredients will also be easy to find. Just take note, as some facial masks need to be kept refrigerated in order to extend the life of the mixture without spoiling. Most homemade facial masks are made from fresh ingredients, making it prone to quick spoilage.

Facial masks are an ideal weekly treat for tired skin weathered by stress and pollution, keeping the face fresh and moisturized all the time. The fresh ingredients will help keep the skin nourished, improve its elasticity and keep it protected from the everyday stresses of the weather. The sun rays and the cold weather can be very harmful to the skin, so it is important to keep the skin always protected. After using the mask, follow up with a natural sun block and moisturizer to keep the skin further protected.

Here is a list of facial mask recipes ideal for all types of skin.

Natural Banana Mask

Ingredients: 1/2 very ripe banana, 1 teaspoon Vitamin E oil, and 1 tablespoon yogurt

Directions: Mash the banana in a bowl and mix in the Vitamin E and yogurt. Apply it on a clean face and leave on for 30 minutes. Rinse with lukewarm water.

Main Ingredient: Banana

*The banana is natural skin moisturizer. Its Vitamin C, B6, and A content help keeps the skin elastic and hydrated while repairing any skin damage.***Moisturizing Orange Mask**

Ingredients: juice from 1 orange, 2 teaspoons dried orange peel, ½ cup oatmeal (steel-cup type), 3 tablespoons plain Greek yogurt, and 2 tablespoons honey

Directions: Gather all the ingredients and pour them in a bowl. Stir until well-combined. The consistency should be thick not runny. Apply the mask on a clean face. Leave on for 30 minutes and rinse with warm water.

Main ingredient: Orange

Oranges, especially its peels, has high vitamin C content. This vitamin is very effective in keeping the skin healthy and eliminating blemishes and dark spots. The citric acid in the acid helps remove excess dirt and oil on the skin. It also dries up acne faster and reduces appearance of pimple marks. The essential oils found in the orange peel also rejuvenate and brighten skin, improve skin color and texture, and improve sagging skin.

Honey Almond Mask

Ingredients: 1 tablespoon honey and 3 almonds

Directions: Soak the almonds in water overnight. Place the soaked almonds in the blender and grind them finely. Remove from blender and transfer to a clean bowl. Slowly add a spoonful of honey into the ground almonds and stir well. Add a few drops of water until a paste is formed. Apply on a clean face and massage on a circular motion. Leave on for 30 minutes before rinsing with warm water and then, cold water.

Main ingredient: almonds

Almonds are rich in vitamin E. It protects the skin from the sun's ultraviolet rays, nourishes the skin to keep it moisturized and supple, and slows down aging.

Peach Facial Mask

Ingredients: 1 egg white and 1 very ripe peach

Directions: Put the peach in a food processor and puree until thick. Whisk the egg white until stiff peaks form and gently fold in the pureed peach. Apply to the face and neck. Leave on for 20-25 minutes and rinse with warm water.

Main ingredient: peach

Peach does wonders for tired and dried skin. Its high Vitamin C and A contents keep the skin healthy and refreshed. It moisturizes dry skin, regenerates skin cells, and brightens the complexion.

Pore Tightener Mask

Ingredients: 1 egg, 1 tablespoon organic honey, 1 teaspoon finely chopped fresh mint leaves, and 1 teaspoon crushed dried chamomile flowers

Directions: In a small bowl, whisk the egg and honey together. Add the rest of the ingredients and stir well. Massage on clean skin and let dry. Wash off with warm water and then, a splash of cold water.

Main ingredients: chamomile and mint leaves

Chamomile flowers contain healing, cleansing, and moisturizing properties which make it a really effective skin care treatment. It soothes sunburn, eliminates acne scars, hastens healing of minor wounds, reduces dark eye circles, and stops premature aging. The mint leaves' astringent properties soothe itching and infected skin, strengthen the facial skin tissue, and reduces sebum production. It also cleanses the skin to prevent clogged pores and promote clearer skin.

Cocoa Coffee Rejuvenating Mask

Ingredients: 5 tablespoons cocoa powder, 5 tablespoons freshly ground coffee, 8 tablespoons Greek yogurt, and 2 tablespoons raw honey

Directions: Slightly warm the honey in a small bowl. Add in the rest of the ingredients and mix well. Apply on the face and let set for 15 minutes. Rinse well.

Main ingredient: Coffee

Coffee increases blood circulation on the skin to give a rosy, healthy glow. It also tightens the skin and fights premature skin aging. The smell also revitalizes the soul and senses.

Rejuvenating Pumpkin Mask

Ingredients: ½ cup pumpkin pulp, 2 medium eggs, 1 teaspoon honey, 2 teaspoon almond milk, 2 teaspoon apple cider vinegar (substitute with cranberry juice if you have oily skin)

Directions: Place the cut up pumpkin pieces in a food

processor or blender to puree into a thick paste. Add in the honey and almond milk. Next, add in the apple cider vinegar, or cranberry juice if the skin is oily. Mix everything together until thoroughly blended. Apply the mask on the face and leave on for 15 to 20 minutes. Rinse thoroughly with cold water then apply moisturizer afterwards.

Main ingredient: Pumpkin

Pumpkin is known to be rich in vitamin A when consumed. But when applied topically on the skin, it helps soften fine lines, calm pimple breakouts and brighten complexion.

Egg Whites and Yogurt Mask

Ingredients: 2 egg whites, 2 tablespoons plain unflavored yogurt

Directions: Separate the egg whites from the yolk and place in a bowl. Add in the yogurt and mix together thoroughly. Apply on the face and leave on for a few minutes before rinsing with warm water.

Main ingredient: egg whites

Egg white is best known to remedy oily skin. It draws out the oil from the skin and tightens the pores. It also helps get rid of white heads which is actually caused by oil blocking the pores of the skin.

Homemade Clay Mask

Ingredients: ½ teaspoon green clay, 1 ½ tablespoon aloe vera, ½ teaspoon kaolin clay, 1 tablespoon rosewater, 2 drops rose essential oil

Directions: Mix the green and kaolin clay together before

adding in the rest of the ingredients. Apply thinly on the face and leave on for 10 to 15 minutes before rinsing. Pat the skin dry and apply moisturizer. Keep the mixture refrigerated and it can last up to four weeks.

Main ingredient: kaolin clay

Kaolin clay has long been used in facial beauty products because of its nourishing, purifying and healing effects. It is chemical free and is ideal for oily skin.

Milk Powder Face Mask

Ingredients: 1 tablespoon milk powder, 1 tablespoon honey, 1 tablespoon lemon juice, ½ tablespoon almond oil

Directions: Place all the ingredients in a bowl and mix well. Apply a thin layer of the mixture on the face and other body parts. Let it stay for 15 minutes before rinsing.

Main ingredient: milk powder

Cleopatra, well known queen on Egypt, was known to bathe in milk to make her skin soft, supple and radiant. Milk contains lactic acid that helps in the exfoliation of the skin. Milk is also used to reduce pigmentation, discoloration and wrinkles.

Italian Salad Mask

Ingredients: 1 ripe tomato, ½ tablespoon olive oil

Directions: Mash the ripe tomato until it is watery and pulpy. Add the olive oil. Apply on the face and leave for 10 minutes. Don't leave it on the face for more than this time as it may sting.

Main ingredient: tomato

Tomato is well known to have Vitamin C and antioxidants that can make the skin healthy. This mixture is best for skin lightening because of the tomato and moisturizing because of the olive oil.

Chapter 6: Facial Masks and Scrubs for Oily and Acne-Prone Skin

What most people will look for in a face scrub is its ability to gently remove dirt and excess oil without causing any irritation. Those who have acne problems are usually not recommended to scrub their face often as it might further aggravate the problem. However, there are some types of face scrubs that are safe and its components have anti-acne properties that will be beneficial for the skin. If the skin is oily, a gentle home face scrub will be beneficial to keep oil and sebum from clogging the pores.

There are several ingredients that are safe and effective if a person is troubled with oil and acne. One is oatmeal, which is an effective cleanser oil remover. For oily skin, there's lemon juice and red clay. Coffee grounds and tea tree help get rid of harmful bacteria that contribute to acne production. Honey is also an effective facial cleanser as well as anti-inflammatory agent for troublesome acne.

A good facial scrub may contain one or two of these ingredients, and not necessarily all of them. Thus, below is a list of facial mask recipes ideal for those with oily and acne prone skin.

Citrus Yogurt Mask

Ingredients: 1 cup yogurt (plain, not non-fat), 1 teaspoon carrot juice, 1 teaspoon fresh orange juice, and 1 teaspoon fresh lemon juice

Directions: Combine all the ingredients in a bowl. Apply to clean face and leave on for 10 minutes. Wipe off with washcloth dipped in warm water. Follow up rinse with cold water.

Main ingredient: orange and lemon juice

Orange and lemon juice contains a lot of nutrients that keep the skin fresh and young-looking. It effectively protects again free radical damage too. Lemon juice also lightens skin and reduces appearance of acne scars. The acid in these citrus juices mildly cleanses and removes excess oil.

Strawberry Mask

Ingredients: 9 strawberries and 3 tablespoons honey

Directions: Place the strawberries in a bowl and roughly mash with a fork. Add the honey and combine well. Apply on the face and leave on for several minutes before rinsing.

Main ingredient: strawberries

Strawberries effectively cleanses the skin while tightening the pores and sloughing off dead skin cells. It also regulates oil production and reduces appearance of acne.

Plum Almond Mask

Ingredients: 5-6 plums and 1 teaspoon almond oil

Directions: Boil the plums in water until soft. Transfer to a bowl and mash. Add the almond oil and combine well. Massage on the face for several minutes and rinse when dry.

Main ingredient: plums

Full of vitamin E , plums effectively prevent wrinkles and loss of skin elasticity. It also lightens dark spots, freckles, and other skin discoloration.

Peppermint Mask

Ingredients: 2 teaspoon dried peppermint, 2 teaspoon dried lavender, ½ cup almonds, 1/2 cup rolled oats, and ½ cups white cosmetic clay

Directions: Place the oats, almonds, and dried herbs in the spice grinder or high powered food processor. Grind into a very fine powder. Transfer the ground mixture in a bowl and add in the cosmetic clay. Mix well. Get a handful of the mixture and slowly add several drops of water to turn it into paste. Apply on the skin and leave on for 10 to 15 minutes. Rinse with warm water.

Main ingredient: peppermint

Peppermint reduces sebum production without drying out the skin. It also balances the skin's pH levels to prevent acne, pimples, and blackheads.

Creamy Thyme Face Mask

Ingredients: 1 tablespoon sour cream, 1 tablespoon fresh thyme leaves, 1 teaspoon unfiltered raw honey, ½ teaspoon lemon juice

Directions: Put all the ingredients in a blender or food processor. Process until the thyme leaves is shredded in tiny pieces. Apply the mask to a clean face and leave on for 10-15 minutes. Rinse well with warm water.

Main ingredient: thyme

When it comes to healing acne, thyme's properties greatly rival the benzoyl peroxide. It cleanses the skin, removes deep-seated dirt, and reduces any swelling. Importantly, it doesn't have any side effects compared to other pimple-fight chemical product.

Veggie Facial Mask

Ingredients: 1 teaspoon parsley, 1 teaspoon cucumber (unpeeled), and 1 teaspoon yogurt

Directions: Place all the ingredients in a blender. Process until creamy. Massage on clean skin and leave on for 15 minutes. Rinse with lukewarm water.

Main ingredient: cucumber

Cucumber naturally reduces appearance of dark eye circles and puffy eyes. It also soothes the skin, improves the skin's complexion, fades facial scars, and minimizes pore size.

Tomato Oatmeal Mask

Ingredients: 1 teaspoon rolled oats, 1 teaspoon lemon juice, and 1 ripe tomato

Directions: Place all the ingredients in a blender. Process until a fine mush is achieved. Apply on clean skin and leave on for 30 minutes. Wipe off with a damp washcloth before rinsing with cold water.

Main ingredient: tomato

Tomatoes delay skin aging and appearance of wrinkles. Full of vitamin C, it gets rid of blackheads, dries out acne, and heal acne-related wounds and infections.

Breakout Busting Mask

Ingredients: 3 drops fresh lemon juice, 1 teaspoon raw honey, and 1 teaspoon ground cloves

Directions: Mix all the ingredients in a small bowl. Apply on the face and leave to dry. Rinse with lukewarm water.

Main ingredient: ground clove

Ground clove contains anti-inflammatory properties that reduce acne swelling. It also evens out complexion and exfoliates the skin to bring out a wonderful glow.

Bay Leaf Clay Mask

Ingredients: 5 dried bay leaves, 4 tablespoons French green clay, and 1 cup distilled water

Directions: Boil the water and put in the bay leaves. Let steep for 10 minutes and let cool Discard the leaves and add in the clay. Once a paste is formed, apply on the face and allow to dry. Rinse with warm water.

Main ingredient: bay leaves

Bay leaves liven up tired and stressed skin. It reduces appearances of fine line and acne outbreaks. Its healing properties heal insect bites and stings and bacterial infections.

Carrot Face Mask

Ingredients: 2 to 3 medium-sized carrots, 4 ½ tablespoons honey

Directions: Boil the carrots until soft. Mash the carrots using a food processor or a mashing utensil. Add the honey and mix well together. Refrigerate the mixture for at least 10 minutes. Apply on the face and leave it on for at least 10 minutes. Rinse with cold water. Keep the leftover mixture refrigerated.

Main ingredient: carrots

Carrots are great sources of Vitamin A, Vitamin C and potassium. These are antioxidants that help repair damaged skin tissues, making it look more youthful. Carrots are very good for the skin whether eaten or applied. The honey contains enzymes, minerals, vitamins and amino acids that supply nutrients to the skin - making it healthy.

Honey-Papaya Mask

Ingredients: 1/3 cup ripe papaya, ¼ cup honey, 1/3 cup cocoa, 3 tablespoons of heavy cream, 3 tablespoons oatmeal powder

Directions: Place all ingredients in a bowl and mix together until well blended. Apply mixture on the face and leave it on for at least 10 minutes. Rinse the face with warm water.

Main ingredient: papaya, honey

This mask is ideal for oily and acne prone skin. It also has anti-aging effects. It helps get rid of blemishes and impurities while balancing the skin's pH levels. It helps nourish the skin leaving it soft and radiant looking.

Green Tea Scrub Mask

Ingredients: 2 green tea bags, 1 tablespoon sugar, ½

tablespoon lemon juice, oatmeal flakes

Directions: Make a cup of green tea using 2 tea bags. Place hot water on a cup and leave the tea bags for about an hour. Remove the bags and then add the sugar and lemon juice. Put the mixture in the refrigerator. This mixture should be good for about a week. When needed, take 2 tablespoons of the tea mixture and soak 1 tablespoon of rough oatmeal flakes in it. Massage onto face in a circular motion. Leave on for at least 20 minutes before rinsing. Moisturize skin afterwards.

Main ingredient: green tea

Green tea has amazing antioxidant properties, meaning it is excellent for cell regeneration. It helps the skin produce new cells more effectively, making the skin look youthful.

Orange Peel Mask

Ingredients: orange peels, 1 tablespoon rose water, 1 tablespoon raw milk (use apple cider vinegar instead of milk if skin is extremely oily)

Directions: Put the orange peels out in the sun to dry. When dried, grind the peels in a mixer and add the rose water and milk. Apply onto face and leave on for 15 minutes before washing off.

Main ingredient: orange peels

This is an excellent mixture for treating acne and lightening tan removals. The orange peels can help soothe sun burnt skin.

Chapter 7: Facial Mask for Dry and Sensitive Skin

Pollution, harmful sun rays, and stress - people are exposed to these on a daily basis while the skin receives all the damaging effects. With the rapid changing of the weather from extreme heat to chilling cold, more people find their skin becoming dry and sensitive. The winter season, most specially, can do so much damage to the skin, making it blotchy and flaky. That's why it is important to keep the skin, specially the face, extra clean and hydrated.

How do you know if you have sensitive skin? People who have sensitive skin easily react to harsh skin care products and to changes in the weather and environment. Common skin reactions include having skin bumps, pustules and skin erosions. People who have sensitive skin can have very dry skin that easily flush and blush. Having sensitive skin is mostly caused by environmental factors, but sometimes genetics, age, gender and race can play a part.

One of the best ways to gently rid the skin of impurities while sealing in moisture is with the use of facial masks. One advantage of making your own mask is that you are assured that you are using fresh and high quality ingredients. People with sensitive skin easily react to chemicals. Most store-bought facial masks are chockfull of chemicals. This is done in order to extend the shelf life of the product.

Homemade facial masks may not last as long as store-bough products but they work even better in locking in moisture and maintaining the softness and glow longer. The chemicals in most store-bought products can cause an even greater damage to the skin in the long run compared to the natural, organic ingredients used in homemade face masks.

Here's a list of homemade facial mask recipes for dry and sensitive skin.

For Dry Skin

Lemon Egg Mask

Ingredients: 1 egg yolk, 1 teaspoon turmeric powder, and 1 teaspoons olive oil

Directions: Whisk the egg yolk and add in the turmeric. Add the olive oil slowly. Mix well. Apply the mask on face and neck. Leave on the face until dry. Wipe off with a damp, warm washcloth. Rinse with cold water.

Main ingredient: egg yolk

Egg yolks contain zinc, vitamin A, vitamin B2, and vitamin B3 that help reduce swelling, heal minute cracks and wounds, and soften and moisturize skin. Constant application of this facial mask also brightens the skin and evens skin tone.

Flour Mayo Mask

Ingredients: 4 teaspoons gram flour, 2 teaspoons wheat flour, 1 tablespoon mayonnaise and 4 tablespoons honey

Directions: Place all in the ingredients in the blender. Process until thick. Apply on the face and leave on for 20 minutes before rinsing with cool water.

Main ingredient: mayonnaise

Mayonnaise contains eggs, soybean oil, and vinegar which are quite beneficial for the skin. The eggs and soybean oil effectively moisturizes skin and while the vinegar encourages skin cell regeneration to make skin brighter.

Strawberry and Papaya Mask

Ingredients: 1 peach (cooked), 2 fresh strawberries (large), ½ very ripe papaya, 1 tablespoon oatmeal, and 1 teaspoon honey (organic)

Directions: Place all the fruits in a bowl. Mash and mix together. Stir in the oatmeal and until thick paste is formed. Apply on the face and leave on for 15 minutes. Rinse with warm water.

Main ingredients: strawberry and papaya

Strawberries contain vitamin C, natural exfoliants, and antioxidants which tighten pores, remove impurities, soften skin. It also lightens age spots and freckles. Papaya keeps the skin hydrated and supple because it doesn't contain any sodium. It also slows down skin aging.

Fennel Seed Mask

Ingredients: 1 tablespoon fennel seeds, 1 tablespoon honey, and 1 tablespoon oatmeal

Directions: Steep the fennel seeds in ½ cup of boiling water for 10 minutes. Strain the liquid and let cool. Grind the oatmeal using a food processor. Add the ground oatmeal to the fennel tea. Mix in the honey. Apply on the face and rinse after 20 minutes with tepid and cold water.

Main ingredient: Fennel seed

Fennel effectively regulates the skin's moisture level to make the skin supple and moisturized. It also stimulates the blood circulation which make the skin toned, elastic, and smooth.

Aloe Vera Mask

Ingredients: 1 teaspoon aloe vera juice, ½ teaspoon jojoba oil, 2 tablespoons of green clay, 1 drop lavender oil, and 1 drop bergamot oil

Directions: Combine all the ingredients and stir well. Add a few drops of water to make a paste. Apply on the face and leave on for 15 minutes. Rinse off with warm water.

Main ingredients: aloe vera juice

Aloe vera moisturizes the skin without making the skin overly greasy. It also reduces skin inflammation, reduces fine lines, and minimizes facial scarring.

Yummy Chocolate Mask

Ingredients: 1 plain dark chocolate bar, 1 cup milk, 3 tablespoons salt

Directions: Gradually melt the chocolate bar in a double boiler. Add in the milk and salt. Stir the mixture thoroughly and let cool to room temperature. Apply a thin layer on the face (and neck area if preferred) and let it dry for 10 to 15 minutes. Rinse with warm water.

Main ingredients: dark chocolate

Dark chocolate contains compounds that help revitalize dry and tired skin.

Turmeric Mask

Ingredients: 1 teaspoon turmeric, 1 tablespoon flour, 2 tablespoons coconut oil or olive oil

Directions: Combine all ingredients together in a bowl and mix well. Apply the mixture on the face and leave it on for at least 10 to 15 minutes. Rinse with warm water.

Main ingredients: turmeric

The turmeric spice helps restore dry, flaky and dull-looking skin. When combined with oil, it acts as a brightening agent that helps the skin look radiant and glowing.

Milk Mask

Ingredients: 1 teaspoon powdered milk, 1 tablespoon honey, 1 tablespoon aloe vera gel

Directions: Combine all ingredients together in a bowl and mix well. Apply the mixture on the face and leave it on for at least 10 to 15 minutes. Rinse with warm water.

Main ingredients: milk, Aloe Vera

Milk has been used since the ancient times to whiten and moisturize skin. It is particularly helpful for dry skin that has already started to crack and flake. Aloe Vera helps to repair damage skin.

Rose Petal Mask

Ingredients: 1 tablespoon yogurt, 1 tablespoon honey, 2 tablespoons rose water, fresh rose petals

Directions: Grind the fresh rose petals and place in a bowl.

Add in the yogurt and the honey. Mix all the ingredients together until it forms a smooth paste. Apply on the face and leave on for at least 20 minutes. Rinse with cold water.

Main ingredients: rose water

This mixture is perfect for those with combination to dry skin as well as an oily t-zone. Roses have long been used by cosmetic companies on their products because of their benefits on the skin. It has anti-inflammatory properties that can soothe an irritated skin. It is also a rich source of antioxidants that help in skin regeneration.

For Sensitive Skin

Avocado Yogurt Mask

Ingredients: ½ cup yogurt (plain, not non-fat), ¼ cup honey, and 1 very ripe avocado

Directions: Slice the avocado open. Remove the seed and remove the flesh of the avocado. Place the avocado meat in the bowl and mash it in chunks. Mix in the yogurt and honey. Stir well. Apply the mask on a clean face and leave for 30 minutes. Rinse off with warm water.

Main ingredient: avocado and yogurt

The avocado fruit is rich in vitamin A, vitamin D, and vitamin E. All these vitamins help keep the skin healthy, young, and moisturized. The yogurt contains various enzymes, zinc and protein that helps cleanse and soften skin.

Rose Clay Mask

Ingredients: 1 tablespoon rose clay, 1 drop rose oil, 2 teaspoons avocado oil, 1 drop Roman chamomile oil

Directions: Combine all the ingredients in a bowl. Add a few drops of water to create a paste. Apply on clean face and let dry. Rinse off with warm water and, then cold water.

Main ingredient: rose clay

A mild kaolin clay, rose clay gently cleanses and exfoliates the skin by removing dead skin cells and opening clogged pores. It also improves the blood circulation on the face and gives it a rosy, pink glow.

Cornmeal Chamomile Mask

Ingredients: 1 tablespoon freshly brewed chamomile tea, and 1 teaspoon milk powder, and 1 teaspoon cornmeal

Directions: Pour the chamomile tea in a bowl and slowly add in the milk powder. Stir well before adding the cornmeal. Once a paste is formed, apply on the skin and leave on for 10 minutes. Rinse with warm water.

Main ingredient: chamomile tea

Chamomile tea contains antioxidants that prevent acne and future breakouts. It also provides a natural, pinkish glow.

Nutmeg Face Mask

Ingredients: 1 tablespoon raw manuka honey, 1 teaspoon ground nutmeg powder, ½ teaspoon Vitamin E oil (1 capsule)

Directions: Mix all the ingredients together in a bowl until it forms a thick paste. Apply the mixture all over the face, particularly in the problem areas. Leave on for at least 20 minutes, best up to 1 hour. Rinse off with lukewarm water.

Main ingredient: nutmeg

Nutmeg is a powerful ingredient that has anti-inflammatory and soothing properties that help relieve pain and itching. This is especially helpful for acne-prone and sensitive skin. It can gently scrub away impurities from pores to reduce scarring.

Banana and Honey Mask

Ingredients: ½ mashed banana, ½ cup oatmeal, 1 medium egg, ½ tablespoon honey

Directions: Mix all the ingredients together until it forms a thick paste. Massage onto the face in a circular motion. Leave on for at least 15 minutes or until the skin feels firm. Rinse with warm water.

Main ingredient: banana

Bananas contain Vitamin A while the eggs contain lecithin which is a natural skin emollient. The oatmeal is filled with vitamins and minerals that help moisturize and gently cleanse the skin.

Rice Powder Face Scrub

Ingredients: ½ lemon, 2 tablespoons rose water, 1 teaspoon rice powder

Directions: Squeeze the juice from the lemon and add the rose water and rice powder. Mix well until it forms a thick paste. Apply on skin and let it stay for 5 minutes. When dried, gently scrub in a circular motion for 5 minutes. Then let it stay on the face for another 2 minutes before rinsing well with cold water.

Main ingredient: rice powder

Rice powder is excellent for removing dead skin cells. The lemon juice acts as a natural whitening agent on the skin.

Conclusion

Thank you again for purchasing this book!

I hope this book was able to help you make easy and effective body scrubs and facial masks. Remember to choose the mask and body scrub that is most beneficial to your type of skin in order to reap the full benefits derived from the fresh ingredients. Keep the containers airtight and away from moisture and direct sunlight in order to preserve it for future use. Take note of mixtures that need to be refrigerated in order to extend their storage life.

The next step is to experiment further with various natural ingredients. When using fruits for the scrub, it is best to choose a recipe with fruits that are in season so the price will be less in the market. Remember that all the ingredients don't need to be very expensive. Experiment on which body scrub and facial mask is best for you. Most importantly, relax and enjoy every scrub and face mask's scent and the rejuvenating feel that they offer whenever you use them.

Finally, if you enjoyed this book, please take the time to share your thoughts and post a review on Amazon. We do our best to reach out to readers and provide the best value we can. Your positive review will help us achieve that. It'd be greatly appreciated!

Thank you and good luck!

Check Out My Other Books

Below you'll find some of my other popular books that are popular on Amazon and Kindle as well. Simply click on the links below to check them out. Alternatively, you can visit my author page on Amazon to see other work done by me.

Coconut Oil for Easy Weight Loss: A Step by Step Guide for Using Virgin Coconut Oil for Quick and Easy Weight Loss

http://www.amazon.com/Coconut-Oil-Easy-Weight-Loss-ebook/dp/B00JG8H8DE

Superfoods that Kickstart Your Weight Loss Learn How to Use 30 Superfoods to Boost Weight Loss, Immunity and to Live a Healthier Lifestyle

http://www.amazon.com/Superfoods-that-Kickstart-Your-Weight-ebook/dp/B00JNAPM9M

Carrier Oils for Beginners: Discover the Characteristics and Beauty and Health Benefits of Carrier Oils For mixing Aromatherapy Essential Oils

http://www.amazon.com/Carrier-Oils-Beginners-Characteristics-Aromatherapy-ebook/dp/B00K88GI2S

Natural Homemade Cleaning Recipes For Beginners: Essential Oil Recipes For Household Cleaning, Laundry & Toxic Free Living http://www.amazon.com/Natural-Homemade-Cleaning-Recipes-Beginners-ebook/dp/B00K87UBQI

The Best Secrets of Natural Remedies: The Ultimate Guide to Natural Remedies to Prevent and Cure Illnesses, Cold and Flu for Your Family

http://www.amazon.com/Best-Secrets-Natural-Remedies-Illnesses-ebook/dp/B00JNDCOCM

The Hypothyroidism Handbook:An Everyday Guide to Natural Solutions of living with Hypothyroidism including increased energy, lasting weight loss, and general well-being

http://www.amazon.com/Hypothyroidism-Handbook-Solutions-including-increased-ebook/dp/B00JNIGIV0

The Hyperthyroidism Handbook: An Everyday Guide to Natural Solutions of Living with Hyperthyroidism including Weight Gain, Increased Energy and General Well-being

http://www.amazon.com/Hyperthyroidism-Handbook-Solutions-including-Hypothyroidism-ebook/dp/B00JOHU5SM

Essential Oils & Weight Loss for Beginners: Ultimate Guide to Losing Weight, Increasing Energy, Balancing Metabolism & Appetite Using Essential Oils & Aromatherapy

http://www.amazon.com/Essential-Oils-Weight-Loss-Beginners-ebook/dp/B00JOFOWP6

Top Essential Oil Recipes: A Recipe Guide Of Natural, Non-Toxic Aromatherapy & Essential Oils for Healing Common Ailments, Beauty, Stress & Anxiety

http://www.amazon.com/Top-Essential-Oil-Recipes-Aromatherapy-ebook/dp/B00JY434E2

Soap Making For Beginners: A Guide to Making Natural Homemade Soaps from Scratch, Includes Recipes and Step by Step Processes for Making Soaps

http://www.amazon.com/Soap-Making-Beginners-Homemade-Processes-ebook/dp/B00JYKH75I

Body Butters For Beginners: Proven Secrets To Making All Natural Body Butters For Rejuvenating And Hydrating Your Skin

http://www.amazon.com/Body-Butters-Beginners-Rejuvenating-Hydrating-ebook/dp/B00K6LVV6A

Apple Cider Vinegar For Beginners: Proven Secrets Using Apple Cider Vinegar For Health, Weight Loss, and Skin Care

http://www.amazon.com/Apple-Cider-Vinegar-Beginners-Aromatherapy-ebook/dp/B00K6YY6HI

Homemade Body Scrubs & Masks For Beginners: 50 Proven All Natural, Easy Recipes For Body & Facial Masks To Exfoliate Nourish, & Care For Your Skin

http://www.amazon.com/Homemade-Body-Scrubs-Masks-Beginners-ebook/dp/B00K79D4SY

Essential Oils Box Set #1: Essential Oils & Weight Loss For Beginners (Ultimate Guide to Losing Weight, Increasing Energy, Balancing Metabolism & Appetite Using Essential Oils & Aromatherapy) + Top Essential Oil Recipes (A Recipe Guide of Natural, Non-Toxic Aromatherapy & Essential Oils for Healing Common Ailments, Beauty, Stress & Anxiety)

http://www.amazon.com/ESSENTIAL-OILS-BOX-SET-Aromatherapy-ebook/dp/B00K7Q8HRK

Essential Oils Box Set #2: Essential Oils & Weight Loss For Beginners (Ultimate Guide to Losing Weight, Increasing Energy, Balancing Metabolism & Appetite Using Essential Oils & Aromatherapy) + Top Essential Oil Recipes (A Recipe Guide of Natural, Non-Toxic Aromatherapy & Essential Oils for Healing Common Ailments, Beauty, Stress & Anxiety)

http://www.amazon.com/ESSENTIAL-OILS-BOX-SET-Aromatherapy-ebook/dp/B00K7Q8HRK

Box Set#3: Coconut Oil for Easy Weight Loss(A Step by Step Guide for Using Virgin Coconut Oil for Quick and Easy Weight Loss) + Apple Cider Vinegar(Proven Secrets Using Apple Cider Vinegar for Health, Weight Loss, and Skin Care)

http://www.amazon.com/Box-Set-Beginners-Aromatherapy-Essential-ebook/dp/B00K9TEGUW

Box Set #4: Body butters For Beginners(Proven Secrets To Making All Natural Body Butters For Rejuvenating And Hydrating Your Skin) & Top Essential Oil Recipes: A Recipe Guide Of Natural, Non-Toxic Aromatherapy & Essential Oils for Healing Common Ailments, Beauty, Stress & Anxiety http://www.amazon.com/Box-Set-Butters-Beginners-Essential-ebook/dp/B00KA02F4Y

Box Set #5: Soap Making For Beginners(A Guide to Making Natural Homemade Soaps from Scratch, Includes Recipes and Step by Step Processes for Making Soaps) + Homemade Body Scrubs & Masks For Beginners(50 Proven All Natural, Easy Recipes For Body Scrub & Facial Masks To Efoliate, Nourish, & Care For Your Skin)

http://www.amazon.com/Box-Set-Beginners-Homemade-Recipes-ebook/dp/B00K9U3I2I

Box Set #6: Body Butters for Beginners (Proven Secrets To Making All Natural Body Butters For Rejuvenating And Hydrating Your Skin) +Homemade Body Scrubs & Masks For Beginners(50 Proven All Natural, Easy Recipes For Body Scrub & Facial Masks To Exfoliate, Nourish, & Care For Your Skin)

http://www.amazon.com/Box-Set-Beginners-Exfoliating-Moisturizing-ebook/dp/B00K9U3Y4O

Box Set #7: TOP ESSENTIAL OILS(A Recipe Guide Of Natural, Non-Toxic Aromatherapy & Essential Oils For Healing, Common Ailments, Beauty, Stress & Anxiety) & THE BEST SECRETS OF NATURAL REMEDIES(The Ultimate Guide to Natural Remedies to Prevent and Cure Illnesses, Cold and Flu for Your Family)

http://www.amazon.com/BOX-SET-Essential-Recipes-Remedies-ebook/dp/B00K9WPMQG

Box Set #8: NATURAL HOMEMADE CLEANING RECIPES FOR BEGINNERS (Essential Oil Recipes for Household Cleaning, Laundry & Toxic Free Living) + TOP ESSENTIAL OILS(A Recipe Guide Of Natural, Non-Toxic Aromatherapy & Essential Oils For Healing, Common Ailments, Beauty, Stress & Anxiety)

http://www.amazon.com/BOX-SET-Beginners-Essential-Aromatherapy-ebook/dp/B00KAMNGBS

Box Set #9: Essential Oils & Weight Loss for Beginners (Ultimate Guide to Losing Weight, Increasing Energy, Balancing Metabolism & Appetite Using Essential Oils & Aromatherapy) + Carrier Oils for Beginners (Discover the Characteristics and Beauty and Health Benefits of Carrier Oils for Mixing Aromatherapy Essential Oils)

http://www.amazon.com/BOX-SET-Essential-Beginners-Aromatherapy-ebook/dp/B00KAODL6Q

BOX SET #10: THE HYPERTHYROIDISM HANDBOOK (An Everyday Guide to Natural Solutions of Living with Hyperthyroidism including Weight Gain, Increased Energy and General Well-being) + THE HYPOTHYROIDISM HANDBOOK (Everyday Guide to Natural Solutions of Living With Hypothyroidism Including Increased Energy, Lasting Weight Loss, and General Well-Being)

http://www.amazon.com/BOX-SET-10-Hyperthyroidism-Hypothyroidism-ebook/dp/B00KAKMSBY

BOX SET #11: CARRIER OILS FOR BEGINNERS (Discover the Characteristics and Beauty and Health Benefits of Carrier Oils for Mixing Aromatherapy Essential Oils) + Essential

Oils & Aromatherapy for Beginners (Secrets to Beauty, Health and Weight Loss Using Proven Essential Oil and Aromatherapy Recipes

http://www.amazon.com/BOX-SET-Beginners-Essential-Aromatherapy-ebook/dp/B00KAONEQ8

BOX SET 12: ESSENTIAL OILS & WEIGHT LOSS FOR BEGINNERS: (Ultimate Guide to Losing Weight, Increasing Energy, Balancing Metabolism & Appetite Using Essential Oils & Aromatherapy) + TOP ESSENTIAL OIL RECIPES (A Recipe Guide of Natural, Non-Toxic Aromatherapy & Essential Oils for Healing Common Ailments, Beauty, Stress & Anxiety) + CARRIER OILS FOR BEGINNERS (Discover the Characteristics & Beauty & Health Benefits of Carrier Oils for Mixing Aromatherapy Essential Oils) + ESSENTIAL OILS & AROMATHERAPY FOR BEGINNERS (Secrets to Beauty & weight Loss Using Proven Essential Oil & Aromatherapy Recipes) + NATURAL HOMEMADE CLEANING RECIPES FOR BEGINNERS (Essential Oil Recipes for Household Cleaning, Laundry & Toxic Free Living)

http://www.amazon.com/BOX-SET-12-Essential-Aromatherapy-ebook/dp/B00KCBCHE4

BOX SET #13: SUPERFOODS THAT KICKSTART YOUR WEIGHT LOSS (Learn How to Use 30 Superfoods to Boost Weight Loss, Immunity and to Live a Healthier Lifestyle) + ESSENTIAL OILS & AROMATHERAPY FOR BEGINNERS (Secrets to Beauty, Health and Weight Loss Using Proven Essential Oil and Aromatherapy Recipes) + BODY BUTTERS FOR BEGINNERS (Proven Secrets To Making All Natural

Body Butters For Rejuvenating And Hydrating Your Skin) + SOAP MAKING FOR BEGINNERS (A Guide to Making Natural Homemade Soaps from Scratch, Includes Recipes and Step by Step Processes for Making Soaps) + HOMEMADE BODY SCRUBS FOR BEGINNERS (50 Proven All Natural, Easy Recipes For Body Scrub & Facial Masks To Exfoliate, Nourish, & Care For Your Skin)

http://www.amazon.com/BOX-SET-Superfoods-Kickstart-Aromatherapy-ebook/dp/B00KC8G6DK/

BOX SET 14: Essential Oils & Weight Loss for Beginners (Ultimate Guide to Losing Weight, Increasing Energy, Balancing Metabolism & Appetite Using Essential Oils & Aromatherapy) + Apple Cider Vinegar for Beginners (Proven Secrets Using Apple Cider Vinegar for Health, Weight Loss, and Skin Care) + Body Butters For Beginners (Proven Secrets To Making All Natural Body Butters For Rejuvenating And Hydrating Your Skin)
+ Homemade Body Scrubs & Masks for Beginners (50 Proven All Natural, Easy Recipes for Body Scrub & Facial Masks to Exfoliate, Nourish, & Care for Your Skin) + Coconut Oil for Easy Weight Loss (A Step by Step Guide for Using Virgin Coconut Oil for Quick and Easy Weight Loss)

http://www.amazon.com/BOX-SET-Essential-Beginners-Aromatherapy-ebook/dp/B00KEDO68U

www.ingramcontent.com/pod-product-compliance
Lightning Source LLC
Chambersburg PA
CBHW071413290526
45789CB00003BA/1265